Fats

by Rhoda Nottridge

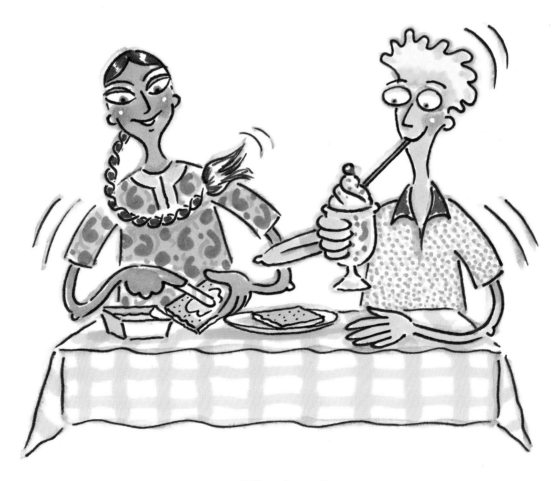

Wayland

— FOOD FACTS FAT —

Additives
Vitamins
Fibre
Sugar
Fats
Proteins

Publishers note

The publishers apologise for the following errors in this book:

Page 10

Lines four to eight of the first paragraph should read:
This kind of fat is often used in processed foods such as cakes and biscuits, because it lasts longer than unsaturated fats.

Lines three and four of the third paragraph should read:
A lot of saturated fat in our diet is bad for our health.

Words printed in **bold** can be found in the glossary on page 30.

First published in 1992 by Wayland (Publishers) Ltd
61 Western Road, Hove, East Sussex, BN3 1JD

British Library Cataloguing in Publication Data

Nottridge, Rhoda
  Fats. – (Food Facts series)
  I. Title II. Series

ISBN 0 7502 0513 X

© Copyright 1992 Wayland (Publishers) Ltd

Series Editor: Kathryn Smith
Designer: Helen White
Artwork: John Yates
Cartoons: Maureen Jackson

Typesetting by White Design
Printed and bound in Belgium by Casterman S.A.

Contents

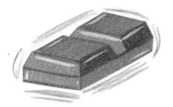

What is fat?

We all need lots of **energy**, especially when we are growing. Fats, which can be found in many foods, are a very rich source of energy. They can give us up to twice as much energy as some other kinds of foods. We need to eat some fat to have the energy just to stay alive!

BELOW We need some fat in our diet to give us energy for life! Body fats also provide our bodies with warmth against the cold.

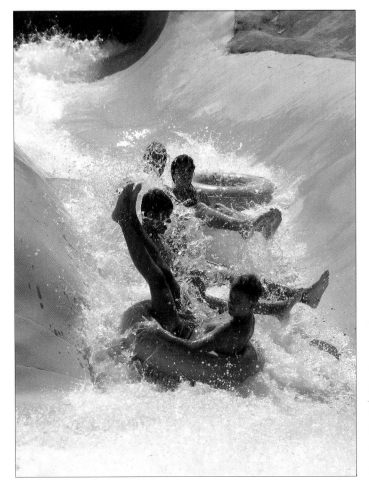

Fats provide our bodies with warmth. They also cushion delicate parts of our bodies so that they are less likely to get damaged. Fats also contain **vitamins** A, D, E and K, and some important **minerals**.

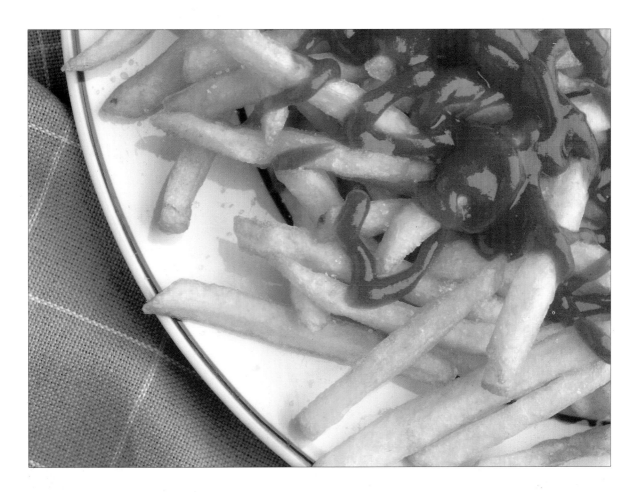

These are all needed to keep our bodies healthy.

Fats add flavour and texture to food, making things more tempting to eat. A meal which contains fats also helps to make us feel full for longer, because fat stays in our stomach for quite a long time.

There are solid fats, such as butter, and liquid fats like cooking oils. We can actually see fats in some food. In meat such as bacon, the fats are the white bits in between the red meat. On fried foods like chips, you can see the grease because it makes the food shiny.

In foods like milk and cheese, it is not so easy to spot these kind of fats. As you cannot see them easily they are called hidden or invisible fats. Quite a lot of food you eat may contain fats that are invisible to the eye. Many of your favourite foods, such as chocolate, nuts, ice-cream, biscuits, cakes, sauces, salad

ABOVE Chips which have been fried in oil contain at least 5 per cent fat. You can see it glistening on their surface.

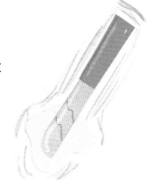

creams and other **processed** foods, all contain hidden fats.

Nearly all liquid fats are kinds of vegetable oil. These oils come from the seeds of particular plants. Hard fats like butter come from dairy products or from the meat of animals.

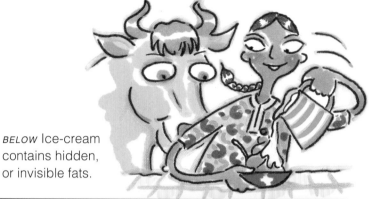

BELOW Ice-cream contains hidden, or invisible fats.

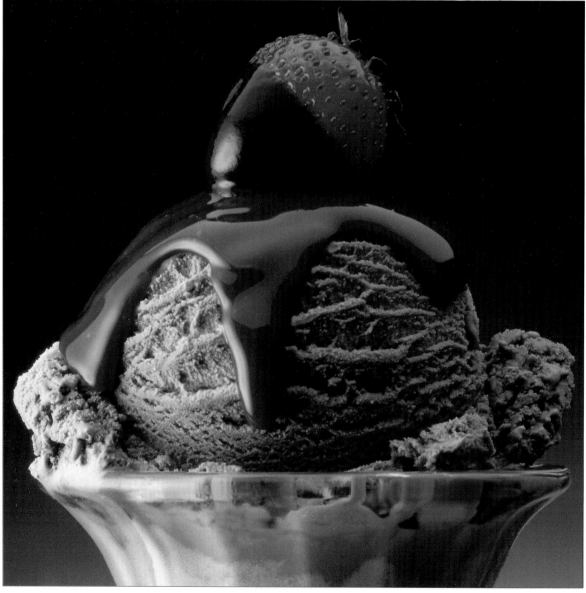

Science Corner

You cannot always tell if a food contains fat, simply by looking at it. Here is an experiment to help you to tell which foods contain fat.

You will need:
2 pieces of greaseproof paper.
1 slice of tomato.
1 piece of cheese.

1. Lay out two pieces of greaseproof paper.
2. Gently rub a piece of cheese on one piece of the paper.
3. Now gently rub a slice of tomato on the other piece of paper.
4. Remove the slices of cheese and tomato. Leave the papers to dry.
5. When the papers are dry, there will be a grease stain where the cheese lay and no grease stain where the tomato was. This shows that cheese is a fatty food and that tomato does not contain any fat. You can try this experiment with any food to see if it contains fat.

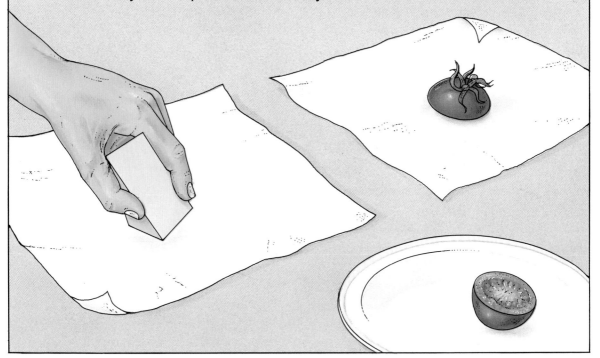

Fat Facts

Although we usually just use the word 'fat', there are in fact several different types. Our bodies use each one differently. We need to be able to tell the difference between each type, if we want to look after our health.

BELOW Vegetable oils, animal fats, dairy products and fruit and nuts all contain varying amounts of different types of fat.

The diagram on page 9 shows how fats and oils can be divided into groups. There are two main types of fats and oils. These are called **saturated** and **unsaturated** fats and oils. Saturated fats come mainly from animals.

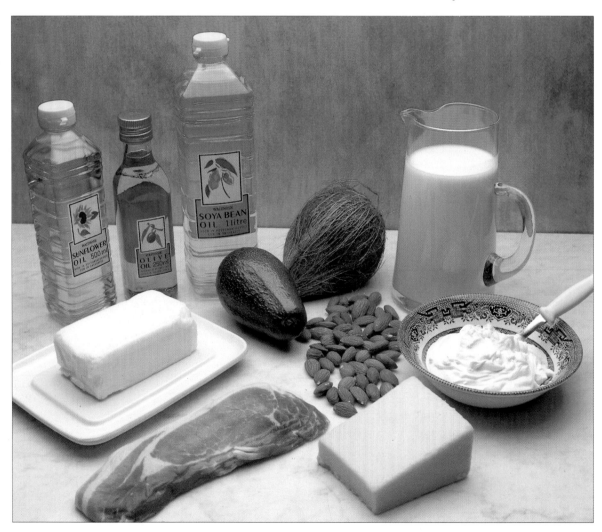

FATS

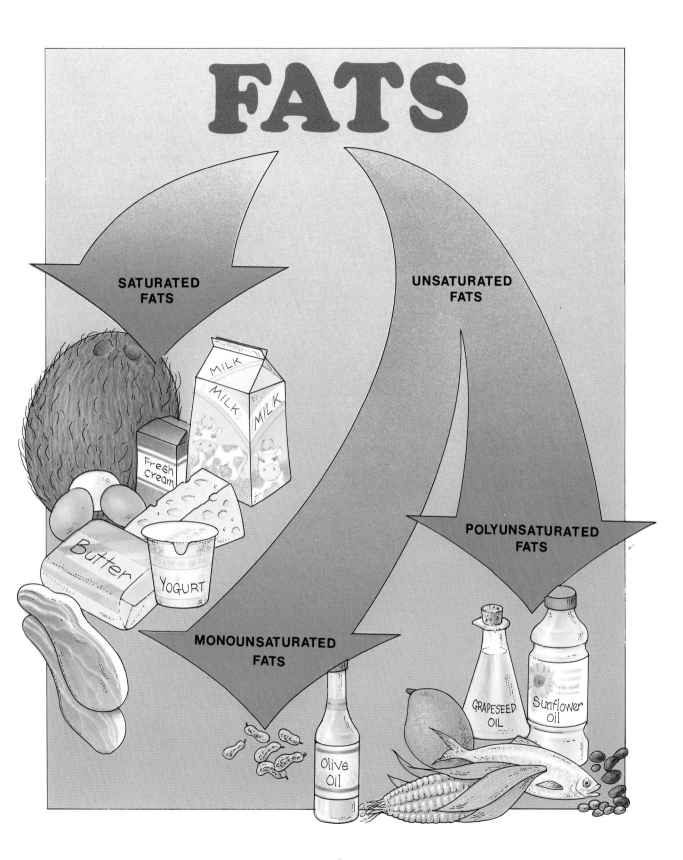

SATURATED FATS

UNSATURATED FATS

POLYUNSATURATED FATS

MONOUNSATURATED FATS

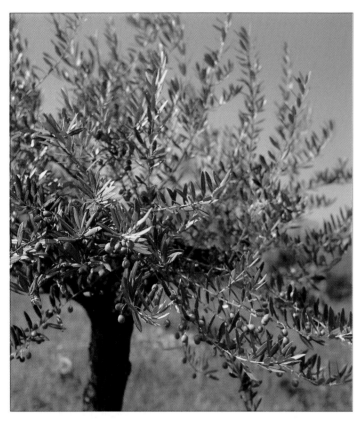

plants, such as their seeds, fruit or vegetables. Hundreds of plants have seeds which contain some oil, but only a dozen of these are commonly used to make vegetable oils. These include sunflower, soya and grapeseed oils.

Healthy Options

How much of what we eat of each kind of fat affects our health. A lot of unsaturated fat in our diet is bad for our health. Eating polyunsaturated and monounsaturated fats instead is better for us.

How can we tell which type of fat we are eating? We can make a good guess simply by

Saturated fats include milk and milk products, eggs, and the white fat that can be seen on meat. This kind of fat is often used in processed foods such as cakes and biscuits, because it lasts longer than saturated fats. Although nearly all saturated fats come from animals, coconut oil and palm oils also happen to be high in saturated fats.

Unsaturated fats can be divided up further into **poly-unsaturated** and **mono-unsaturated** fats. These fats usually come from parts of

ABOVE Olive oil, which is high in monounsaturated fat, comes from the fruit of the olive tree. After picking, the fruit is pressed to extract the oil.

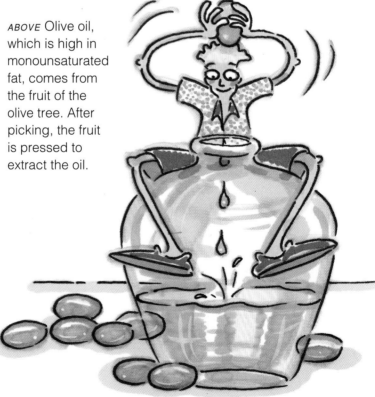

looking at how hard, soft or liquid a fat or oil is. At room temperature corn oil is a liquid. It is high in polyunsaturates, making it an unsaturated fat. At the same temperature beef dripping is hard. This is a highly saturated fat. So the harder a fat, the more likely it is to be high in saturates. The softer a fat is, the more likely it is to be unsaturated.

As with all rules, there are always a couple of exceptions.

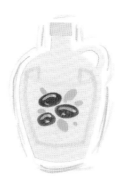

BELOW Oil from sunflower seeds is high in poly-unsaturated fat.

Olive oil is a kind of mono-unsaturated fat (unsaturated fat), which behaves differently. In a warm room, it is a liquid, whilst it turns cloudy and mushy if it is kept in the cold. Also some fats are processed at food factories, so that what we buy as a hard fat may once have been a liquid fat. The best way to be sure of what we are eating is to look at the label of a food product, where all the ingredients are listed.

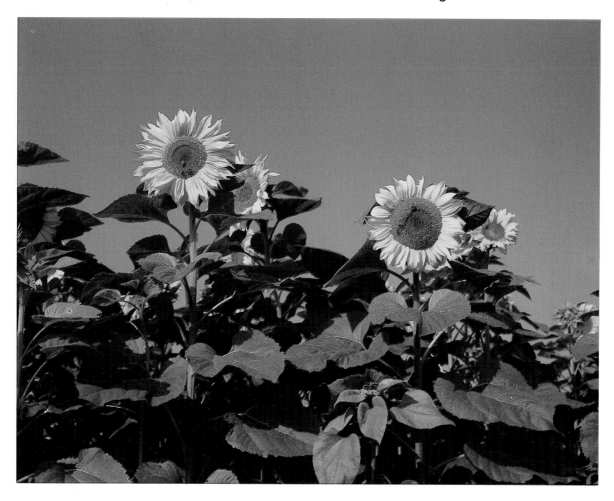

Science Corner
A polyunsaturated salad: Quick Bean Bonanza
This tasty salad uses polyunsaturated oil.

Ingredients:
1 x (approximately) 200 g
can of kidney beans
½ green pepper
1 apple
2 sticks of celery

For the salad dressing:
2 teaspoons sunflower oil
1 teaspoon lemon juice
½ teaspoon French seed mustard
pinch of black pepper

Method
First prepare the salad dressing.
1. Put the oil, lemon juice, mustard and black pepper into a clean
   screw-top jar.
2. Make sure the lid is screwed on securely, then shake the mixture
   up and down until the oil and lemon are mixed up together.

For the salad:
1. Drain and rinse the kidney beans and put in a large bowl.
2. Carefully wash the celery, apple and pepper. Chop the celery into
   fine slices. Take the core out of the apple and the middle out of the
   pepper and throw them away. Then chop up the apple and pepper
   into small pieces.
3. Mix them all together in a bowl.
4. Add the salad dressing and mix in.
   Your salad is ready to serve!

The heart of the matter

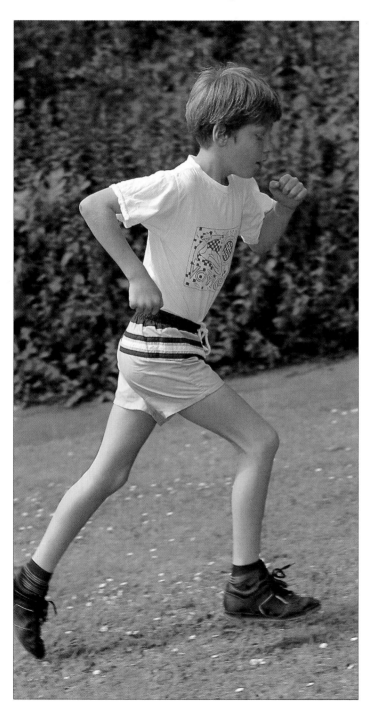

The heart has to work day and night to continuously pump blood around every part of the body. It is actually just a muscle, the size of a fist. It pumps the blood carrying the oxygen that we breathe in around our bodies. At the same time it collects the **carbon dioxide** which the body returns, and pumps it back into the lungs, so we can breathe it out.

Our blood is carried to and from the heart through a network of tubes, called **arteries**. Fats are needed in our blood to help it to flow round the body.

If we have too much fat in our blood, it starts to stick to the inside of the arteries. This narrows the tubes and affects the flow of blood to the heart. This narrowing of the tubes starves the heart of the oxygen it needs to work properly, so that a heart attack may occur.

LEFT Jogging increases the speed at which our hearts beat, causing blood to be pumped around our bodies at a faster rate. This reduces the chance of fats in the blood sticking to the artery walls.

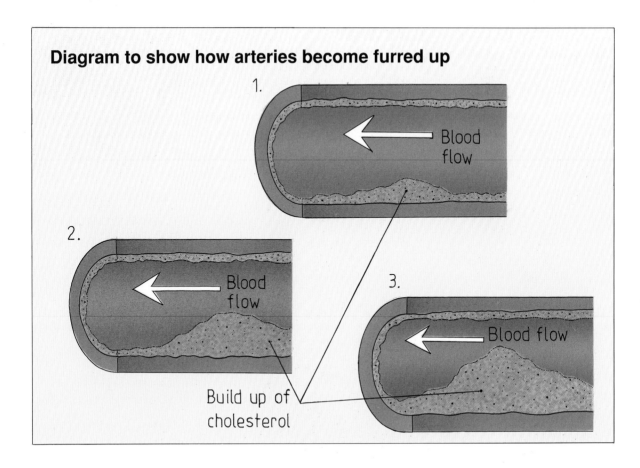

Diagram to show how arteries become furred up

1.

Blood flow

2.

Blood flow

3.

Blood flow

Build up of cholesterol

Heart attacks are also caused when an artery tube gets blocked by a **blood clot**. Sticky blood containing too much fat can cause a clot to build up in a tube.

There are different types of fat in our blood. One of these is called **cholesterol**. It is a very important fat which our bodies need. We can get cholesterol from eating saturated fats which come from animal products or by getting our bodies to make it for us, mainly in our livers.

ABOVE A diagram to show how cholesterol furs up the arteries. If our bodies contain too much cholesterol, it gradually sticks to the insides of the arteries, narrowing them.

If our bodies have too much cholesterol, it is normally turned into waste. Some people's bodies are not able to do this. The level of cholesterol in their blood stays high. Because there is too much fat going round the arteries, it gradually sticks to the tubes, narrowing them.

To find out if someone may be likely to have heart disease, they can have their blood tested to see how much cholesterol their blood contains. (Other factors such as smoking and not exercising also affect how likely someone is to get heart disease.) If people have a lot of fat in their blood, they need to cut down the amount of fat that they eat.

They also have to make sure that the fats that they do eat are high in polyunsaturates rather than high in saturates. This is because the fats such as cholesterol which are most likely to stick to the arteries come from saturated fats.

We all need to change to eating more polyunsaturated fats instead of saturated fats. It has been shown that the Inuit of Greenland and fishermen in Japan are less likely to get heart problems compared to other people. This is because although their diets are quite high in fat, they eat a lot of fish which is high in polyunsaturates. It has also been found that people whose diet includes a lot of olive oil, such as in Italy, are also less likely to get heart disease, because olive oil is a monounsaturated fat.

We need to make sure that we take enough exercise, so that our blood gets pumped through the arteries and there is less chance of sticky fats in the blood sticking to the sides of the tubes.

BELOW The Inuit of Greenland eat a diet of raw Arctic Char (fish), which is high in polyunsaturated fat.

In the Western world, we all eat too much of all kinds of fat anyway. Nearly half the energy we take from food comes from fat. That means that we eat about 90 g of fat each day. The amount of fat we eat should only be a third of our diet, which is around 70 g a day.

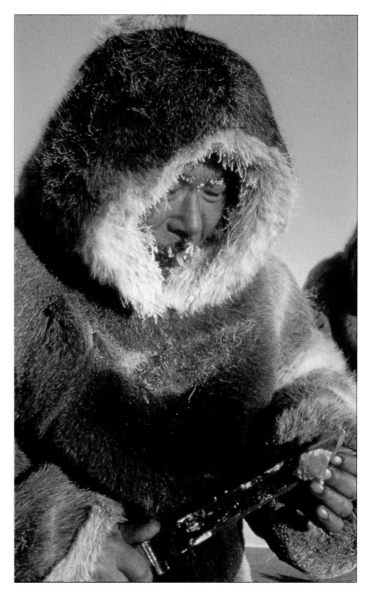

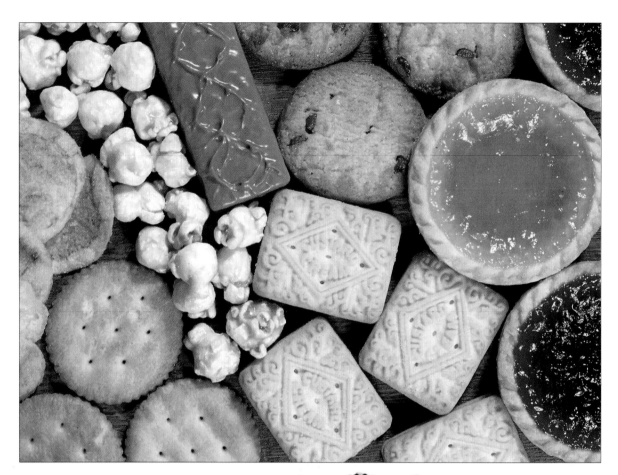

ABOVE
In the Western world we eat far too many fatty foods; about 90 g of fat a day. We should only eat about 70 g of fat each day to remain healthy.

You can exercise to keep your heart fit and healthy. This will give you stamina, so that you don't get out of breath and tired so easily. Exercises which increase your stamina include jogging or running, skipping, cycling, swimming and badminton.

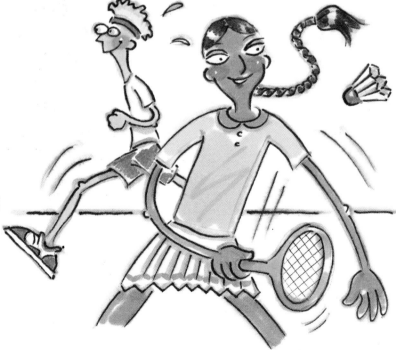

Jog for joy!

Jogging means running at a slow, comfortable pace, breathing regularly. Try to jog on soft ground such as grass rather than on a hard surface such as concrete. Make sure you wear training or running shoes which cushion your feet. Before starting a jog, you need to do some warm-up exercises first. You can do this by just bending and stretching every part of your body in turn, as if you were stretching during a huge yawn.

Have a healthy heart!

Here's a programme to slowly increase your stamina. Each week follow the training programme, doing the amount of exercise suggested three times a week. By the time you get to the sixth week, you will have built up enough stamina to be able to jog for twenty minutes. If you feel any pain or discomfort during jogging, stop immediately and talk to your sports teacher about it.

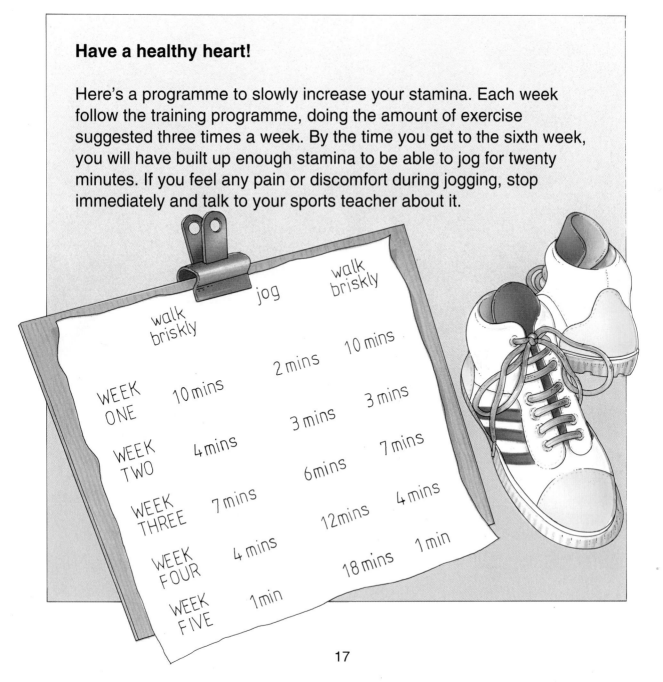

	walk briskly	jog	walk briskly
WEEK ONE	10 mins	2 mins	10 mins
WEEK TWO	4 mins	3 mins	3 mins
WEEK THREE	7 mins	6 mins	7 mins
WEEK FOUR	4 mins	12 mins	4 mins
WEEK FIVE	1 min	18 mins	1 min

Quiz

Do you eat too much fat?
Read the questions and write down the number you score for each
question on a piece of paper.

1. *What type of milk do you drink?*   **score**

gold top	3
silver top	2
semi-skimmed	1
skimmed	0

2. *How often do you eat fried foods, such as chips, bhajias,
samosas or fried rice?*

every day	3
once or twice a week	2
less than once a week	1
hardly ever or never	0

3. *How often do your eat chocolates, cakes and biscuits?*

every day	3
once or twice a week	2
less than once a week	1
hardly ever or never	0

4. *How often do you eat cheese?*

every day	3
once or twice a week	2
less than once a week	1
hardly ever or never	0

5. *How much fat such as butter or margarine do you spread on bread, toast or chapattis?*   **score**

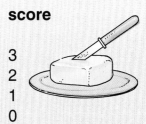

a thick layer   3
a medium amount   2
a thin scrape   1
none at all   0

6. *How often do you eat crisps or nuts?*

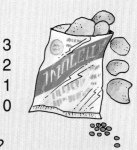

every day   3
once or twice a week   2
less than once a week   1
hardly ever or never   0

7. *How often do you eat sausages, meat pies or burgers?*

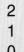
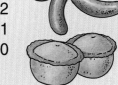

every day   3
once or twice a week   2
less than once a week   1
hardly ever or never   0

Now add up your score.

If you scored 14 or more:
You are probably eating too many fatty foods. Try to cut down on fried foods and fatty snacks. Instead, eat more fresh fruit and vegetables and make sure you take plenty of exercise.

If you score between 7 and 13:
You eat a reasonable amount of fatty foods but you should take care to make sure that you are aware of which foods are less fatty.

If you score 7 or below:
Well done! You have a diet which is low in fat. Providing the food you eat is varied you should be feeling fit and healthy.

Choosing fats

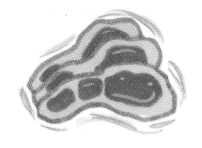

Too much meat?

We can control how much fat we eat by choosing our diet carefully. If we eat meat, then liver, kidney, salami, bacon, pies and pasties tend to all be very fatty. White meat such as chicken and turkey are less fatty, or we may prefer to cut out meat altogether from our diets.

BELOW White meats such as chicken have a lower fat content than red meat and many processed meat products.

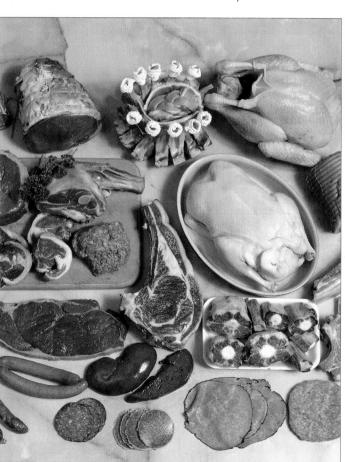

Choosing cheeses

Cheeses are often high in fat. The best way to cut down on this kind of fat is to change cheeses. Cheese such as Cheddar or blue cheese are high in fat. Brie and Edam contain less and cottage cheese is a very low-fat cheese.

Is butter better?

It takes the cream from nearly five litres of milk to make a 250 g pack of butter. As cream is very high in fat, so is butter. Butter is one of the oldest natural dairy products in the world and has been made for centuries. It contains vitamins A and D and contains no additives apart from salt.

Margarine and spreads

Margarine is made from either a mixture of animal and vegetable oils or just from vegetable oils. Most margarines contain the same amount of fat as butter, but the ones made with sunflower or soya bean oil are better for our health because they are high in polyunsaturates.

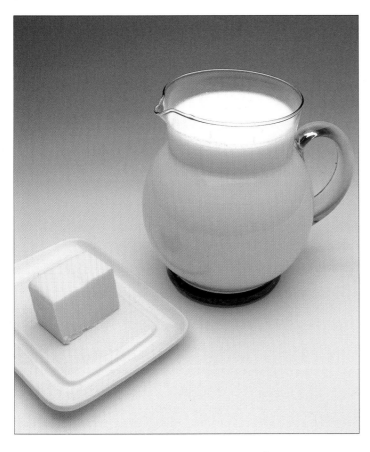

healthy growth of teeth and bones of teenagers.

There is a choice of type of milk you can buy. There is whole, semi-skimmed and skimmed milk. Whole milk has had nothing added to it and nothing taken away. It contains the same amount of fat as when it left the cow. It is suitable for young children who need all the goodness and fat (although it is too rich for small babies).

Semi-skimmed milk has less than half the fat of whole milk because most of the cream has been removed. Although it contains half the fat, it has nearly all the minerals and vitamins of whole milk.

To be called margarine, a product has to be at least 80 per cent fat. There are now a lot of spreads which are much lower in fat, containing as little as 20 per cent. They are useful for spreading but cannot be used for cooking.

Which milk?
Milk is an excellent drink which contains proteins, vitamins and minerals. One of the minerals it contains is calcium, which we all need. It is particularly important for the

ABOVE It takes the cream from this much full fat, or whole milk to make a piece of butter this size!

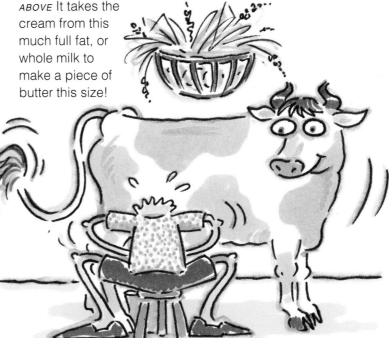

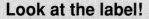

Look at the label!
Look at labels on your favourite foods. You'll probably be surprised at how many foods contain 'hidden' fats.

1. Does the food contain any fats?
2. What different names are the fats given?
3. Do any of the other ingredients contain fat as well?

INGREDIENTS
FLOUR, SUGAR, VEGETABLE OIL, AND HYDROGENATED VEGETABLE FAT AND ANIMAL FAT, PARTIALLY INVERTED SUGAR SYRUP, MALT EXTRACT, SALT, RAISING AGENTS, (SODIUM BICARBONATE, AMMONIUM BICARBONATE).

Semi-skimmed milk is not suitable for young children but it is a healthy choice for the rest of the family.

Skimmed milk has almost all the fat removed from it. It is ideal for people who are trying to lose weight. It is not suitable for children under five. It does not contain all the vitamins, such as Vitamin A, that we get from fatty milks. For this reason, semi-skimmed or whole milk are a better choice for the family and especially for children.

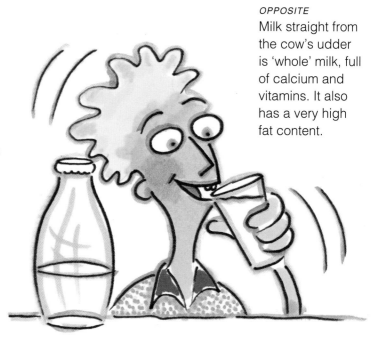

OPPOSITE
Milk straight from the cow's udder is 'whole' milk, full of calcium and vitamins. It also has a very high fat content.

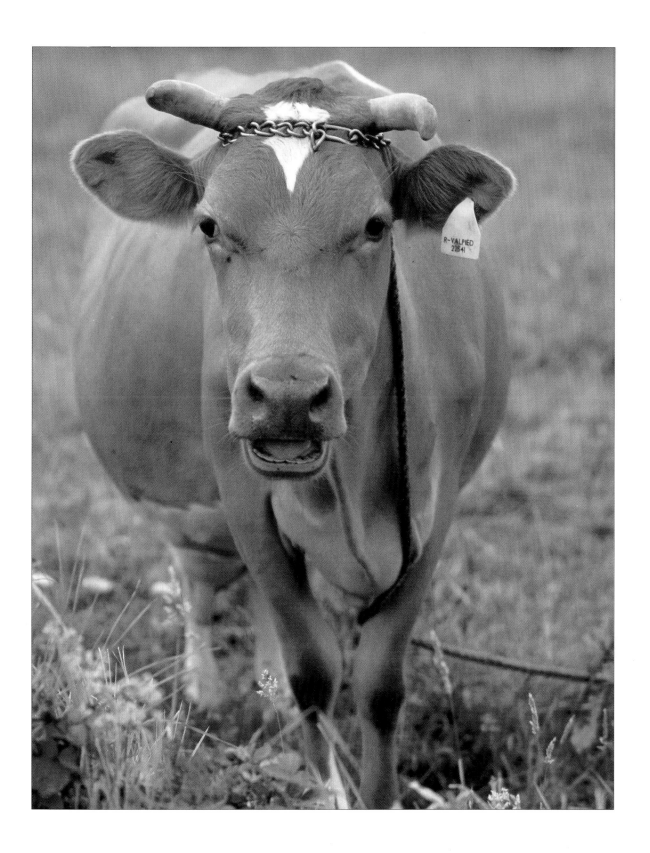

Science Corner

Strawberry Shake
Drinks can be just as nice with semi-skimmed milk once you have got used to it. Try this recipe for a less fatty milkshake.

You will need:
350 ml chilled semi-skimmed milk
2 x 150 g cartons of low-fat strawberry yoghurt
a few fresh strawberries if available

1. Pour the yoghurt into a bowl and add the milk.
2. Use a whisk or fork to mix the two together.
3. Pour into glasses and decorate with a strawberry on top.
4. Serve immediately.

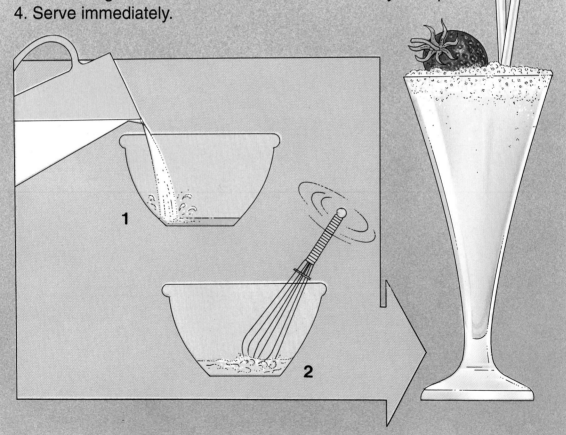

Too fat, too thin ?

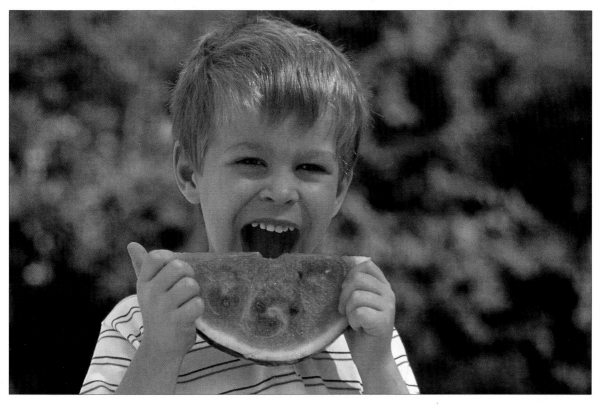

ABOVE We should all eat plenty of fresh fruit and vegetables, which have a high water, vitamin, mineral and fibre content, and eat fewer fatty, sugary foods.

Young people need to get plenty of energy from their food as they are still growing. We all need to have diets which are varied and a balanced mixture of foods. We should eat plenty of fresh fruit, vegetables and cereals and not too much sugar or fatty foods.

Some people are overweight and this makes it harder for their hearts to work. It is not healthy to be overweight. It usually means a person has developed bad eating habits and is not getting enough exercise.

One way for someone who is overweight to thin down is to slowly start to get fit. The other thing they need to change are their eating habits. Too many fatty foods and too much sugar in the diet will cause weight gain.

Quick dieting methods are not worth trying and can be harmful to your health.

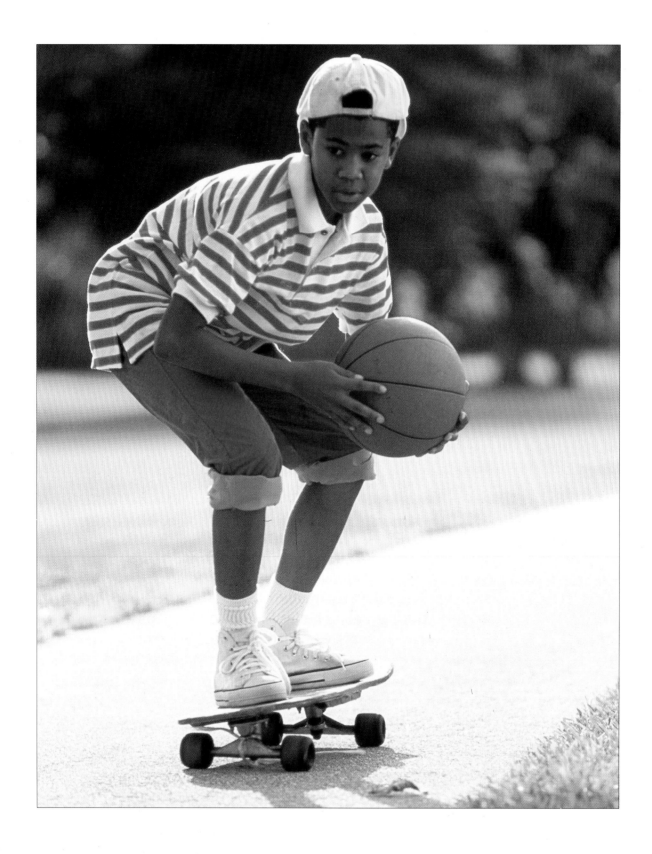

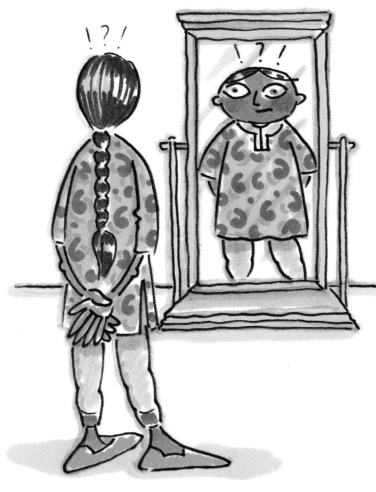

Although it is very important to have a healthy diet and take plenty of exercise, it is also important not to become too worried by your weight.

Girls in particular tend to worry that they are too fat and they try to stop themselves from eating. They may have an idea that they are too fat when they are not really fat at all. They begin to starve themselves and can become seriously ill.

Another eating problem is that some people eat too much to try to cheer themselves up when they are unhappy. If this becomes a habit they feel bad about it and may even make themselves sick.

People can be helped with both these problems, which are very serious. It is important that if you, a friend or relative have an eating problem that you tell someone about it. Talk to a doctor, teacher or someone who you trust about the problem.

The most important way to keep fit and healthy is to take plenty of exercise and eat a balanced diet. This means plenty of fibre foods such as cereals and pulses, wholemeal bread and pasta and plenty of fresh fruit and vegetables and a little less of the fatty foods!

OPPOSITE
Regular exercise will help you to keep your body trim and healthy.

If someone feels they need to slim, they should talk to their doctor or a health education teacher about how to slim and develop sensible eating habits.

Many young people worry that they look too fat or too thin. When we grow our bodies change shape. It is not always easy to accept the new shape! Sometimes people put on weight when they are growing and then lose it when they get taller.

Eat less fats!

Here are some top tips to help you cut down your intake of fats:

1. Cut down on the number of fried foods you eat. Choose grilled or steamed food instead of fried.
2. Eat less meat and cut off the fat and any skin.
3. Spread butter, margarine or ghee (a kind of butter) only very thinly or change to a low-fat spread.
4. On desserts, use a low fat yoghurt instead of cream, evaporated and condensed milk or use half yoghurt mixed with cream.
5. Cut down on eating biscuits, chocolates and savoury snacks.
6. Change to semi-skimmed milk.
7. Choose cheeses which are lower in fat such as Edam, Gouda, Brie, Camembert or cottage cheese.

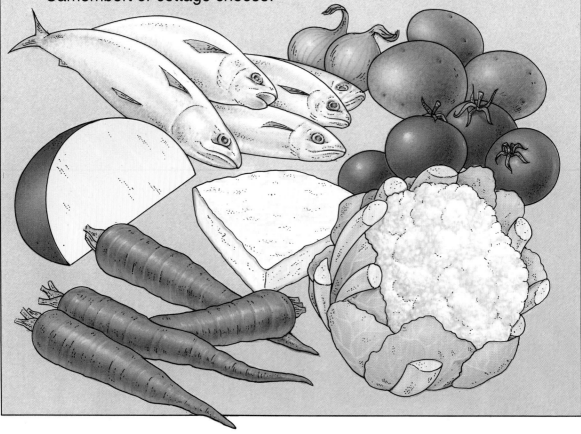

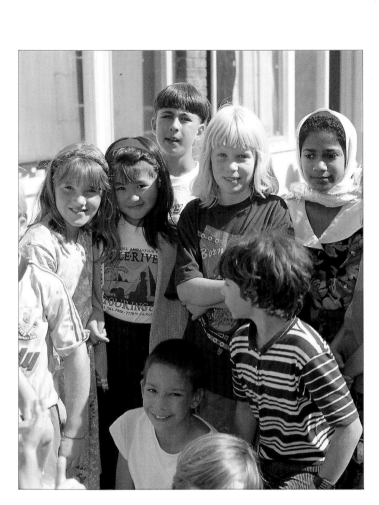

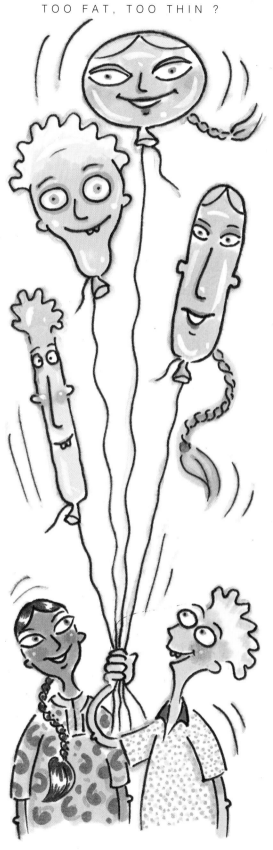

Fill up with fibre!
Just because you're cutting down on fats, it doesn't mean you have to eat less! You can fill up by eating more **fibre**.

Here's how:
1. Eat more wholemeal bread, pasta and potatoes.
2. Eat high-fibre breakfast cereals or porridge or muesli.
3. Instead of meat, eat more beans, lentils or brown rice.
4. Eat more fresh fruit and vegetables.

ABOVE
Shape and size vary vastly between different people. Do not worry about your body shape. As long as you eat a balanced diet and exercise regularly, then you are the right shape for you.

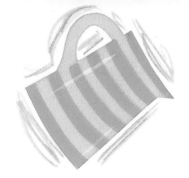

Glossary

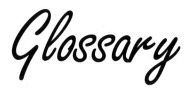

Arteries   The thick-walled tubes that take blood to the heart and to parts of the body.

Blood clot   When blood sticks together in an artery and forms a lump which blocks the tube.

Carbon dioxide   One of the several gases in the air we breathe.

Cholesterol   A type of fat which helps blood flow round our bodies.

Diet   Our diet is made up of the things we eat.

Energy   This is made in your muscles by a reaction between the food we eat and the chemicals in our bodies.

Fatty acids   A chemical name for kinds of fats.

Fibre   A substance found in food such as cereals, that fills you up and helps your digestive system to work.

Food manufacturers   Factories that make processed food.

Heart attack   When the heart stops beating, such as when a blood clot prevents blood flowing properly round the heart.

Minerals   Tiny amounts of substances found in some foods which are important for our health.

Monounsaturated fat   An unsaturated fat which can be found in foods such as olive oil, avocado and peanuts.

Polyunsaturated fat   An unsaturated fat which is found in foods such as vegetable oils.

Processed   When a food has been changed by going through a process at a factory, such as being frozen.

Protein   An essential part of our diet which is found in food such as meat, milk and nuts.

Saturated fat   The kind of fat in meat and dairy products which is usually solid.

Stamina   The strength which we can build up by exercising our heart and lungs.

Unsaturated fat   The kind of fat which is liquid or soft and normally comes from vegetables.

Vitamins   Small amounts of substances found in some foods which are very important for our health.

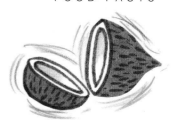

Books to read

Diet and Health by Ida Weekes (Wayland, 1991)

Exercise and Fitness by Brian Ward (Franklin Watts, 1988)

Focus on Dairy Produce by Richard Clark (Wayland, 1985)

Health and Food by Dorothy Baldwin (Wayland, 1987)

Meat by Elizabeth Clark (Wayland, 1989)

Milk by Annabelle Dixon (A & C Black, 1987)

You and your Fitness and Health by Kate Fraser and Judy Tatchell (Usborne, 1986)

You and your Food by Judy Tatchell et al (Usborne, 1985)

Vegetables and Oils by Jacqueline Dineen (Young Library, 1987)

Picture Acknowledgements

Bryan and Cherry Alexander 15; Bruce Coleman 4, 11, 23; Eye Ubiquitous 10, 13, 29; Science Photo Library 16; Wayland Picture Library 8, 21; Zefa 5, 6, 25, 26.

Index

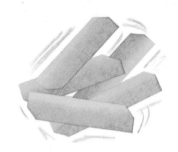